RANJOT SINGH CHAHAL

7-Day Weight Loss Diet Plan

Recipes, Tips, and Motivation for a Healthier You

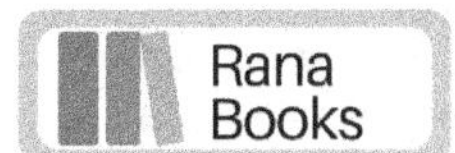
Rana Books

Contents

Introduction

The introduction serves as the opening section of any discussion or written piece, providing a brief overview of the topic at hand. In the context of weight loss, it is crucial to establish a foundation for understanding the importance of a balanced diet and the significance of setting realistic goals.

Weight loss is a complex and multifaceted journey that involves various factors, including dietary choices, physical activity, and mental well-being. In this introduction, it is essential to set the stage by acknowledging the prevalence of weight-related concerns in contemporary society and the various approaches individuals may take to address them.

2. The Importance of a Balanced Diet for Weight Loss:

a. Nutrient Intake:
   A balanced diet is one that provides the body with the necessary nutrients in the right proportions. These include carbohydrates, proteins, fats, vitamins, and minerals. Each nutrient plays a specific role in maintaining bodily functions, and an imbalance can lead to health issues.

b. Energy Balance:
   Weight loss is fundamentally linked to the concept of energy

balance — the relationship between the calories consumed through food and beverages and the calories expended through physical activity and metabolism. A balanced diet ensures that the body receives sufficient energy to function optimally while creating a calorie deficit to promote weight loss.

c. Sustainable and Healthy Approach:
Unlike fad diets that focus on extreme restrictions, a balanced diet promotes a sustainable and long-term approach to weight management. It encourages the consumption of a variety of foods, minimizing the risk of nutritional deficiencies and supporting overall health.

d. Control of Cravings and Hunger:
Balanced meals that include a mix of macronutrients help regulate blood sugar levels, preventing spikes and crashes that can lead to cravings. This, in turn, aids in controlling overall calorie intake and supports weight loss efforts.

3. Setting Realistic Goals:

a. Psychological Aspect:
Weight loss is not only a physical challenge but also a psychological one. Setting realistic goals is crucial for maintaining motivation and preventing frustration. Unrealistic goals can lead to disappointment and may even contribute to the abandonment of healthy habits.

b. Gradual Progress:
Realistic goals involve acknowledging that weight loss is a gradual process. Rapid weight loss often comes with health risks

and is harder to sustain. Setting achievable milestones allows individuals to celebrate small victories and stay committed to their journey.

c. Individualized Approach:
Everyone's body is different, and what works for one person may not work for another. Realistic goals take into account individual differences in metabolism, lifestyle, and preferences. This helps in creating personalized plans that are more likely to be successful.

d. Focus on Health, not just Weight:
While weight loss is a common goal, emphasizing overall health is equally important. Setting goals related to improved energy levels, better sleep, and enhanced mood can contribute to a more holistic and sustainable approach to well-being.

In conclusion, the introduction sets the stage for understanding the critical role of a balanced diet and realistic goal-setting in the context of weight loss. It paves the way for a comprehensive exploration of these topics, considering both physiological and psychological aspects of the weight loss journey.

Day 1: Detox and Cleanse

Detox and cleanse diets have gained popularity in recent years as a way to rid the body of toxins and promote overall health and well-being. These diets often involve eliminating processed foods, caffeine, alcohol, and sugar, and instead focusing on nutrient-rich, whole foods. In this article, we will take a deep dive into Day 1 of a detox and cleanse diet, explaining the benefits and providing examples of each meal and snack.

Breakfast: Green Smoothie Bowl

A green smoothie bowl is a refreshing and nutritious way to kick off your day. It is packed with vitamins, minerals, and antioxidants that help detoxify your body. Here's an example recipe:

Ingredients:
  - 1 cup spinach
  - 1 ripe banana
  - 1/2 cup almond milk (unsweetened)
  - 1 tablespoon chia seeds
  - Toppings: sliced banana, blueberries, granola

Instructions:

1. In a blender, combine spinach, banana, almond milk, and chia seeds.

2. Blend until smooth and creamy.

3. Pour the mixture into a bowl and top with sliced banana, blueberries, and granola.

4. Enjoy your nutrient-rich green smoothie bowl!

Snack: Mixed Nuts

Mixed nuts are a great snack option during a detox and cleanse. They provide healthy fats, fiber, and protein. Here's an example mix:

Ingredients:
- 1/4 cup almonds
- 1/4 cup walnuts
- 1/4 cup cashews
- 1/4 cup pistachios
- Optional: sprinkle of sea salt or cinnamon

Instructions:
1. Combine all the nuts in a bowl.

2. Add a sprinkle of sea salt or cinnamon for flavor.

3. Mix well and portion into snack-sized containers.

4. Carry the containers with you for an easy and nutritious snack on the go.

Lunch: Quinoa Salad

Quinoa is a staple in many detox and cleanse diets due to its high protein and nutrient content. Combined with vegetables and a light dressing, it makes for a satisfying and tasty lunch. Here's an example recipe:

Ingredients:
  - 1 cup cooked quinoa
  - 1 cup mixed vegetables (e.g., cherry tomatoes, cucumber, bell pepper, red onion)
  - Handful of fresh herbs (e.g., parsley, cilantro, mint)
  - Juice of 1 lemon
  - 2 tablespoons olive oil
  - Salt and pepper to taste

Instructions:
  1. In a large bowl, combine cooked quinoa, mixed vegetables, and herbs.
  2. In a separate bowl, whisk together lemon juice, olive oil, salt, and pepper to create the dressing.
  3. Pour the dressing over the quinoa and vegetable mixture and toss until well coated.
  4. Allow the flavors to meld together for a few minutes before serving.

Snack: Fresh Fruit

Fresh fruit is an excellent snack choice for a detox and cleanse day. It is full of vitamins, minerals, and fiber that support digestion and detoxification. Choose a variety of fruits to get a range of nutrients. Some examples include apples, oranges, berries, and melons. Simply wash and cut the fruit into bite-sized pieces, and you have a refreshing snack ready to enjoy.

Dinner: Grilled Vegetables with Baked Salmon

For dinner, focus on incorporating plenty of vegetables and lean proteins. Grilled vegetables and baked salmon make for a delicious and nutritious combination. Here's an example recipe:

Ingredients:
- Assorted vegetables (e.g., zucchini, bell peppers, onions, eggplant)
- 1 salmon fillet
- Olive oil
- Lemon juice
- Salt and pepper
- Herbs of choice (e.g., dill, parsley)

Instructions:
1. Preheat your grill to medium heat.
2. Drizzle the vegetables with olive oil, salt, and pepper, and grill until tender.
3. Place the salmon fillet on a piece of foil and season with salt, pepper, and your preferred herbs.
4. Drizzle the salmon with olive oil and lemon juice, then seal the foil to create a packet.
5. Place the foil packet on the grill and cook for about 15 minutes, or until the salmon is cooked through.
6. Serve the grilled vegetables alongside the baked salmon for a nutritious and satisfying dinner.

Dessert: Yogurt Parfait

A yogurt parfait is a guilt-free dessert option that satisfies your sweet tooth while still providing nutrients. Here's an example recipe:

Ingredients:
- 1 cup Greek yogurt (unsweetened)
- 1/2 cup fresh berries (e.g., strawberries, blueberries)
- 2 tablespoons nuts or seeds of choice (e.g., almonds, chia

seeds)
 - Optional: drizzle of honey or maple syrup for sweetness

Instructions:
 1. In a glass or bowl, layer Greek yogurt, fresh berries, and nuts or seeds.
 2. Repeat the layers until all ingredients are used.
 3. For added sweetness, drizzle a small amount of honey or maple syrup over the top.
 4. Enjoy a satisfying and wholesome dessert without compromising your detox and cleanse goals.

In conclusion, Day 1 of a detox and cleanse diet focuses on nutrient-rich, whole foods that support the body's natural detoxification processes. By incorporating recipes like a green smoothie bowl, mixed nuts, quinoa salad, fresh fruit, grilled vegetables with baked salmon, and a yogurt parfait, you can enjoy a variety of delicious meals and snacks while promoting your overall health and well-being. Remember to stay hydrated throughout the day and listen to your body's needs.

Day 2: High Protein Day

A high protein diet is characterized by consuming an increased amount of protein-rich foods to promote muscle growth, enhance satiety, and support overall health. Day 2 of this high protein meal plan incorporates a variety of delicious and nutritious dishes that are low in fat and high in protein. In this guide, we will explore these meals in detail, including their benefits, nutritional value, and potential alternatives.

Breakfast: Egg White Omelette with Veggies

Starting the day with a nutrient-dense breakfast is essential for an optimal protein intake. An egg white omelette is an excellent choice as it provides a substantial amount of protein while being low in fat and calories. Egg whites are virtually fat-free and contain all the essential amino acids needed for muscle repair and growth.

To make an egg white omelette, whisk together 4-5 egg whites and season with salt and pepper. Cook the egg whites in a non-stick pan and add a variety of veggies such as spinach, bell peppers, and mushrooms. These vegetables not only add flavor and vibrant colors but also contribute additional vitamins, minerals, and dietary fiber to the breakfast.

Snack: Greek Yogurt with Berries

Greek yogurt is a fantastic source of protein, calcium, and probiotics. It offers a creamy and tangy taste while being low in calories. Opting for plain Greek yogurt without added sugars or flavors is recommended to minimize unnecessary additives.

To enjoy this snack, simply combine a cup of Greek yogurt with a handful of fresh berries like strawberries, blueberries, or raspberries. This combination is not only rich in protein but also provides antioxidants, vitamins, and minerals.

Lunch: Grilled Chicken Breast with Steamed Broccoli

Grilled chicken breast is a staple protein source for many athletes and fitness enthusiasts. It is an excellent option as it is low in fat and high in lean protein. Chicken breast is also a great source of B vitamins, magnesium, and selenium.

To prepare this meal, season a chicken breast with herbs, spices, or a marinade of your choice. Grill it until it reaches an internal temperature of 165°F (74°C). Accompany it with a side of steamed broccoli, which not only adds fiber but also contributes vitamins C, K, and A.

Snack: Protein Shake

Protein shakes are convenient and versatile, making them a popular choice for a high protein snack. They are typically made by combining a protein powder with a liquid such as water, milk, or a dairy alternative.

To prepare a protein shake, choose a protein powder that fits your dietary preferences and goals. Whey protein, plant-based protein, or casein protein are common options. Add the desired amount of protein powder to your chosen liquid and mix well. Optional additions like fruits, nut butters, or greens can enhance the taste and nutritional value of the shake.

Dinner: Baked Cod with Asparagus

Fish, such as cod, is an excellent source of high-quality protein and essential omega-3 fatty acids. Baking fish preserves its natural flavors, and the result is a delicious and healthy evening meal.

To prepare baked cod, season the fillet with herbs, spices, or a marinade of your choice. Place it on a baking sheet and bake at 400°F (200°C) for about 12-15 minutes, or until the flesh is opaque and flakes easily. Serve it with a side of asparagus, which adds fiber, vitamins A, C, and K, as well as folate.

Dessert: Protein Brownie

A protein brownie is a satisfying and guilt-free way to end the day on a sweet note. It combines the richness of a classic brownie with the added benefits of high-quality protein.

To make a protein brownie, you will need a protein powder of your choice, along with other ingredients like cocoa powder, almond flour, sweetener, and eggs. Mix the ingredients together and bake until the brownie is firm, yet moist. This dessert provides a balanced mix of macronutrients and satisfies your sweet tooth without the excess sugar and unhealthy fats found in traditional brownies.

Alternative Options:

While the aforementioned meals and snacks provide a solid foundation for a high protein day, it's important to note that individual preferences and dietary restrictions may require modifications. Here are a few alternative options to consider:

- Breakfast: Instead of an egg white omelette, some individuals may prefer a protein-packed smoothie made with protein powder, fruit, and a source of healthy fat like nut butter or avocado.

- Snack: Instead of Greek yogurt, cottage cheese can be a great protein-rich substitute. Combine it with sliced fruits or vegetables for added flavor and nutrients.

- Lunch: Grilled chicken breast is versatile, and it can be substituted with other lean protein sources such as turkey breast, tofu, or tempeh. Pair it with a variety of steamed or roasted vegetables to create a well-rounded meal.

- Snack: If a protein shake is not your preference, you can opt for protein bars or homemade protein balls made with ingredients like oats, nut butter, and protein powder.

- Dinner: If you're not a fan of fish, lean cuts of steak, turkey, or pork can be alternatives. Pair them with a selection of roasted or grilled vegetables for a nutritious meal.

Conclusion:

A high protein day, as exemplified by the meals on Day 2, offers numerous benefits in terms of muscle growth, satiety, and overall health. The examples provided show that incorporating protein-rich foods into your daily meals can be delicious, satisfying, and varied. Whether it's starting the day with an egg white omelette, enjoying a protein shake as a snack, or ending the day with a protein brownie, there are plenty of options to suit different taste preferences and dietary needs. Remember to consult with a healthcare professional or registered dietitian to ensure the meal plan aligns with your specific goals and health conditions.

Day 3: Low Carb Day

Day 3 of the low carb diet focuses on incorporating nutrient-rich foods that are low in carbohydrates. By reducing carb intake, the body is encouraged to burn stored fat for energy instead. This day's meal plan includes a variety of satisfying and delicious dishes that will keep you feeling full and energized throughout the day.

Starting the day with a nutritious and filling breakfast is essential. The Avocado and Smoked Salmon Roll-Up is a perfect choice. Avocado is a great source of healthy fats, while smoked salmon provides a good amount of protein. To make this roll-up, simply spread mashed avocado onto a slice of smoked salmon and roll it up tightly. You can add some lemon juice or herbs for extra flavor.

For a mid-morning snack, Cucumber Slices with Hummus is a refreshing and satisfying option. Cucumbers are low in carbs and high in water content, making them a hydrating choice. Pairing them with hummus adds some protein and healthy fats, making it a balanced snack.

Lunchtime brings a Cauliflower Rice Stir-Fry with Tofu.

Cauliflower rice is a low-carb alternative to regular rice and works well in stir-fry dishes. Tofu adds plant-based protein and absorbs the flavors of the stir-fry sauce. You can customize this dish with your favorite vegetables and seasonings.

Another snack option for the afternoon is a Hard-Boiled Egg. Eggs are an excellent source of protein and healthy fats, essential for a low carb diet. They are also rich in vitamins and minerals that support overall health. A hard-boiled egg is a convenient and portable snack that will keep you satisfied until dinner.

For the evening meal, Zucchini Noodles with Turkey Meatballs is a delicious and low-carb alternative to traditional pasta dishes. Zucchini noodles, or "zoodles," are made by spiralizing zucchini into noodle-like shapes. Turkey meatballs provide a lean source of protein. Top it off with your favorite tomato sauce or pesto for added flavor.

To satisfy your sweet tooth without derailing your low carb diet, enjoy a Sugar-Free Jello for dessert. Regular jello often contains added sugars, which can spike blood sugar levels. However, sugar-free jello provides a sweet treat without the extra carbs and calories. You can even mix in some fresh berries or a dollop of whipped cream for added indulgence.

By following this low carb meal plan on Day 3, you are providing your body with an array of nutrients while keeping carbohydrate intake in check. This approach helps maintain stable blood sugar levels, promotes fat burning, and aids in weight loss. Remember to drink plenty of water throughout the day to stay hydrated and support digestion.

It's worth mentioning that individual dietary needs and preferences may vary. Feel free to adjust portion sizes or swap ingredients according to your requirements and taste preferences. Consulting with a registered dietitian can also provide personalized advice for a low carb diet tailored to your specific needs.

In conclusion, Day 3 of the low carb diet emphasizes incorporating nutrient-rich, low-carb foods for a satisfying and balanced meal plan. The examples provided, such as the Avocado and Smoked Salmon Roll-Up, Cucumber Slices with Hummus, Cauliflower Rice Stir-Fry with Tofu, Hard-Boiled Egg, Zucchini Noodles with Turkey Meatballs, and Sugar-Free Jello, demonstrate the range of delicious and fulfilling options available on a low carb day. With careful planning and creativity, you can enjoy flavorful meals while staying on track with your low carb dietary goals.

Day 4: Plant-Based Day

Day 4: Plant-Based Day is a day dedicated to consuming a variety of delicious and nutritious plant-based meals. By incorporating plant-based ingredients into your diet, you can benefit from the vitamins, minerals, fiber, and phytonutrients found abundantly in fruits, vegetables, legumes, and whole grains. Let's take a closer look at the meals planned for this day.

Breakfast: Vegan Protein Pancakes

Start your day with a stack of Vegan Protein Pancakes. These pancakes are made using plant-based protein sources such as soy, pea, or hemp protein powder, instead of traditional animal-based protein like eggs or dairy. They can be made by combining plant-based milk (such as almond or oat milk), whole wheat flour, protein powder, baking powder, and a sweetener like maple syrup or banana. You can customize your pancakes with topping options like sliced fruits, coconut flakes, or a drizzle of almond butter.

Example: Imagine waking up to a plate of fluffy and nutritious Vegan Protein Pancakes bursting with blueberries, topped with a dollop of dairy-free yogurt and a sprinkle of chia seeds for an added boost of omega-3 fatty acids.

Snack: Almond Butter with Apple Slices

For a mid-morning snack, enjoy the combination of almond butter and apple slices. Almond butter is a rich source of healthy fats, protein, and vitamin E, while apples provide fiber and essential vitamins and minerals. You can either dip the apple slices into the almond butter or spread the almond butter over the apple slices.

Example: Picture yourself savoring the natural sweetness of crisp apple slices dipped in creamy almond butter. The combination provides a perfect balance of flavors and textures, along with a satisfying crunch.

Lunch: Lentil Soup with Whole Grain Bread

For a hearty and nutritious lunch, opt for a warming bowl of Lentil Soup served with a side of whole grain bread. Lentils are an excellent source of plant-based protein, fiber, and various minerals like iron and folate. When cooked together with vegetables, herbs, and spices, they create a delicious and filling soup. Pairing it with whole grain bread adds more fiber and complex carbohydrates to help keep you energized throughout the afternoon.

Example: Imagine enjoying a bowl of aromatic and comforting Lentil Soup, brimming with colorful vegetables such as carrots, celery, and tomatoes. Dip a slice of freshly baked whole grain bread into the soup for a wholesome and satisfying meal.

Snack: Roasted Chickpeas

In the afternoon, indulge in a crunchy and protein-packed snack by roasting chickpeas. Chickpeas, also known as garbanzo beans, are loaded with fiber, plant-based protein, and essential minerals. Coat them in a blend of spices like paprika, cumin, and garlic powder, then bake them until crispy.

Example: Visualize biting into a handful of crispy Roasted Chickpeas, seasoned with smoky paprika, cumin, and a hint of garlic. It's a satisfying and nutritious snack that can be enjoyed on-the-go or while taking a break.

Dinner: Sweet Potato and Black Bean Tacos

For dinner, savor flavorful Sweet Potato and Black Bean Tacos. Sweet potatoes are a great source of vitamins A and C, while black beans provide protein, fiber, and folate. Fill your tortillas with roasted sweet potato chunks, sautéed black beans, and an assortment of fresh vegetables, such as lettuce, tomatoes, onions, and avocados. Top it off with a squeeze of lime juice and a drizzle of a tasty plant-based sauce, like a cilantro-lime crema or avocado cream.

Example: Envision relishing the combination of soft tortillas filled with roasted sweet potatoes, creamy black beans, vibrant vegetables, and a burst of tanginess from freshly squeezed lime juice. The flavors and textures merge together to create a delicious and satisfying taco experience.

Dessert: Vegan Chocolate Pudding

End the day on a sweet note with a guilt-free Vegan Chocolate Pudding. This dessert is made from cocoa powder, plant-based milk, a natural sweetener (such as dates or maple syrup), and a thickening agent (such as cornstarch or chia seeds). Blend the ingredients until smooth and creamy, then refrigerate until set.

You can top it with fresh berries, shredded coconut, or crushed nuts for added texture and flavor.

Example: Imagine indulging in a velvety, chocolatey delight that is both dairy-free and vegan. Each spoonful of the Vegan Chocolate Pudding melts in your mouth, satisfying your sweet tooth while providing the benefits of plant-based ingredients.

By embracing a plant-based day like this, you can explore and enjoy the vast array of flavors and nutrients that exist in plant-based foods. Remember, the examples provided are just a starting point, and you can always customize the meals to suit your preferences and dietary needs.

Day 5: Mediterranean Cuisine

Mediterranean cuisine is known for its fresh ingredients, vibrant flavors, and healthy components. On Day 5 of the Mediterranean cuisine menu, we have a variety of dishes that showcase the essence of this culinary tradition. Let's take a closer look at each meal and explain how they are made.

1. Breakfast: Greek Yogurt Parfait with Granola
   - Greek yogurt is the star of this breakfast. It is thick and creamy, with a tangy flavor.
   - To make the parfait, start by layering Greek yogurt in a glass or bowl. Then add a layer of granola for crunch and sweetness.
   - Repeat the process with additional layers of yogurt and granola.
   - You can customize the parfait by adding fresh fruits like berries or sliced bananas.
   - The combination of protein-packed Greek yogurt and fiber-rich granola makes this a nutritious and satisfying breakfast.

2. Snack: Olives and Cherry Tomatoes
   - Olives are a staple in Mediterranean cuisine, providing a savory and slightly bitter taste.
   - Choose a variety of olives, such as Kalamata or green olives,

for flavor diversity.

- Pair them with cherry tomatoes, which add a burst of juiciness and sweetness to the snack.

- This combination of olives and tomatoes provides a good balance between briny and fresh flavors, making it a simple yet delightful snack.

3. Lunch: Greek Salad with Grilled Chicken

- Greek salad is a classic Mediterranean dish that offers a mix of fresh vegetables and tangy flavors.

- Start by assembling a base of mixed greens or lettuce.

- Add cucumbers, tomatoes, red onions, and bell peppers for crunch and freshness.

- Top it off with feta cheese for its distinctive creamy and salty taste.

- To make it a heartier meal, include grilled chicken, marinated with lemon, olive oil, garlic, and herbs.

- Drizzle the salad with a simple dressing made from olive oil, lemon juice, salt, and pepper.

4. Snack: Hummus with Carrot Sticks

- Hummus is a creamy dip made from chickpeas, tahini, garlic, lemon, and olive oil.

- It's a versatile and protein-rich snack that pairs well with carrot sticks.

- To make hummus, blend together canned chickpeas, tahini, garlic, lemon juice, and olive oil until smooth.

- Season it with salt, pepper, and spices like cumin or paprika for extra flavor.

- Serve the hummus with fresh carrot sticks for a satisfying and nutritious snack.

5. Dinner: Baked Mediterranean Fish with Couscous

   - Baked Mediterranean fish is a delicious and healthy main course.

   - Choose a white fish like cod, halibut, or sea bass for this dish.

   - Marinate the fish with olive oil, garlic, lemon juice, and a blend of Mediterranean herbs such as oregano, thyme, and parsley.

   - Bake the fish until it's tender and flaky.

   - Serve the fish with a side of couscous, which is a quick-cooking grain. Prepare it by boiling water and adding couscous, then covering it and allowing it to absorb the liquid.

   - Season the couscous with salt, pepper, and herbs like mint or cilantro for added freshness.

6. Dessert: Fresh Fruit Salad

   - Mediterranean cuisine emphasizes the use of fresh fruits for desserts.

   - Create a fruit salad by combining a variety of seasonal fruits.

   - Some popular choices include watermelon, oranges, grapes, strawberries, and kiwi.

   - You can enhance the flavor with the addition of a drizzle of honey or a squeeze of lemon juice.

   - This light and refreshing dessert is a perfect way to end the day with a healthy and sweet treat.

Remember, Mediterranean cuisine focuses on using high-quality ingredients and simple preparation methods to bring out the natural flavors. Feel free to adjust the recipes according to your preferences and enjoy the taste of the Mediterranean!

Day 6: Healthy Fat Focus

In today's focus on healthy fats, we have curated a delicious and nutritious meal plan to provide you with examples of how to incorporate healthy fats into your diet throughout the day. Healthy fats are an essential component of a well-balanced diet, as they provide a source of energy, aid in the absorption of fat-soluble vitamins, support brain health, and promote overall satiety. It's important to choose healthy sources of fats, such as monounsaturated and polyunsaturated fats, while limiting saturated and trans fats.

1. Breakfast: Avocado Toast with Poached Egg

Avocados are an excellent source of monounsaturated fats, which have been associated with heart health. For breakfast, you can start your day with a nutritious and filling avocado toast topped with a poached egg. Simply mash half an avocado and spread it on a slice of whole-grain bread. Top it with a poached egg for an additional protein boost. This breakfast provides a good balance of healthy fats, fiber, and protein to keep you satiated throughout the morning.

2. Snack: Almonds

Almonds are a fantastic snack choice when it comes to healthy fats. They contain a good amount of monounsaturated fats, as well as fiber, protein, and various vitamins and minerals. A handful of almonds makes for a convenient and satisfying snack. They can be enjoyed on their own or paired with fresh fruit for added flavor and nutrients.

3. Lunch: Quinoa Bowl with Avocado and Grilled Shrimp

For lunch, we have a delicious and nutritious quinoa bowl packed with healthy fats. Quinoa is a whole grain rich in protein and fiber, while avocado and grilled shrimp add healthy fats to the mix. To make the bowl, cook quinoa according to package instructions and mix it with diced avocado, grilled shrimp, and your choice of vegetables. Drizzle with a light vinaigrette made with olive oil, lemon juice, and herbs for added flavor and healthy fats.

4. Snack: Dark Chocolate Square

Dark chocolate is not only a delicious treat but can also be a source of healthy fats. It's important to choose dark chocolate with a high cocoa content (70% or higher) to reap the benefits. Dark chocolate contains monounsaturated fats as well as antioxidants that may provide various health benefits. Enjoy a square of dark chocolate as an afternoon pick-me-up while satisfying your sweet tooth.

5. Dinner: Grilled Portobello Mushrooms with Feta Cheese

Incorporating healthy fats into your dinners can be both tasty and satisfying. Grilled portobello mushrooms make for a flavor-ful main course, and when paired with feta cheese, they create a satisfying dish rich in healthy fats. Brush the mushrooms with olive oil and your choice of herbs and seasonings, then grill them until tender. Crumble feta cheese on top for a delicious finishing touch.

6. Dessert: Chia Seed Pudding with Berries

For a nutritious and indulgent dessert, chia seed pudding with berries is a fantastic choice. Chia seeds are rich in omega-3 fatty acids, a type of polyunsaturated fat known for its heart-healthy benefits. To make the pudding, soak chia seeds in your choice of milk (such as almond milk or coconut milk) until they expand and turn into a pudding-like consistency. Top it with a handful of fresh berries for added vitamins and minerals.

Incorporating healthy fats into your daily meals can be enjoyable and beneficial for your overall health. The examples provided above demonstrate how you can create a well-rounded meal plan that includes healthy fats in various forms, such as avocado, almonds, quinoa, olive oil, dark chocolate, feta cheese, and chia seeds. Remember to enjoy these foods in moderation as part of a balanced diet and consult with a healthcare professional or nutritionist for personalized advice.

Day 7: Balanced Day

In today's guide, we will explore the concept of a balanced day, focusing on a well-rounded diet that provides essential nutrients throughout the day. We will examine each meal and snack, providing explanations and examples of why they are considered balanced choices. By the end of this guide, you will have a better understanding of how to create a balanced day of eating.

Breakfast: Whole Grain Cereal with Milk and Berries

Starting the day off with a balanced breakfast is essential for providing your body with the energy it needs to kickstart your day. A bowl of whole grain cereal with milk and berries is a perfect choice. Let's break it down:

Whole grain cereal: Opting for whole grain cereal ensures you're getting an adequate amount of fiber which aids in digestion and helps keep you feeling full. Look for cereals with minimal added sugars and a good amount of whole grains.

Milk: Including a source of dairy or dairy alternative, like milk, provides protein, calcium, and other essential nutrients. Milk is an excellent source of calcium, which is crucial for strong bones and teeth.

Berries: Adding fresh or frozen berries to your cereal not only adds natural sweetness but also provides a variety of vitamins, minerals, and antioxidants. Berries are particularly rich in vitamin C and fiber.

Example: A balanced breakfast could consist of a bowl of whole grain cereal (such as oatmeal or bran flakes) topped with a cup of low-fat milk and a handful of mixed berries (such as blueberries, strawberries, or raspberries).

Snack: Trail Mix

A well-balanced snack can help bridge the gap between meals, keeping you energized and satisfied. Trail mix is a convenient and nutritious option that combines various ingredients for a well-rounded snack.

Trail mix typically includes a combination of nuts, seeds, dried fruits, and sometimes chocolate or other sweet additions. This creates a blend of healthy fats, protein, and carbohydrates.

Nuts: Nuts like almonds, walnuts, cashews, or peanuts are packed with healthy fats, fiber, and protein. They contribute to a feeling of fullness and provide essential nutrients like vitamin E and magnesium.

Seeds: Seeds such as pumpkin, sunflower, or chia seeds are rich in omega-3 fatty acids, fiber, and micronutrients. They add a crunchy texture to the mix and provide additional nutritional value.

Dried fruits: Adding dried fruits like raisins, cranberries, or apricots to trail mix provides natural sweetness and a source of fiber, vitamins, and minerals. However, it's important to enjoy dried fruits in moderation due to their higher sugar content.

Example: A balanced trail mix could include a mixture of almonds, pumpkin seeds, dried cranberries, dark chocolate chips, and some air-popped popcorn for added crunch.

Lunch: Grilled Vegetable Wrap

A balanced lunch should incorporate a variety of food groups, including vegetables, protein, and whole grains. A grilled vegetable wrap is an excellent option as it combines various ingredients to create a satisfying and nutritious meal.

Grilled vegetables: Vegetables are a great source of vitamins, minerals, and fiber. Grilling vegetables enhances their natural flavors while keeping them nutrient-dense. Opt for a variety of colorful vegetables like peppers, zucchini, eggplant, and onions.

Protein: Including a source of protein in your wrap is essential for muscle repair and overall satiety. Options like grilled chicken, tofu, or chickpeas can be included.

Whole grain wrap: Choosing a whole grain wrap instead of

refined grains provides more fiber and nutrients. Look for whole grain tortillas or wraps made from whole wheat or other whole grains.

Example: A balanced grilled vegetable wrap could include a whole grain wrap spread with hummus, and filled with grilled vegetables (such as bell peppers, zucchini, and onions), fresh spinach leaves, and grilled chicken or tofu for protein.

Snack: Greek Yogurt with Honey

Having a balanced snack in the afternoon can help maintain energy levels and prevent overeating during dinner. Greek yogurt with honey is a nutritious choice that combines protein, probiotics, and natural sweetness.

Greek yogurt: Greek yogurt is an excellent source of protein and calcium, and it contains probiotics that promote good gut health. Opt for plain, unsweetened Greek yogurt to avoid added sugars.

Honey: Adding a drizzle of honey to your Greek yogurt provides natural sweetness without relying on refined sugars. Honey also contains antioxidants and has antimicrobial properties.

Example: A balanced afternoon snack could consist of a small container of plain Greek yogurt topped with a drizzle of honey and a handful of mixed nuts for extra crunch.

Dinner: Lean Beef Stir-Fry with Brown Rice

Dinner should be well-balanced, satisfying, and provide a variety of essential nutrients. A lean beef stir-fry with brown rice fits the bill, incorporating protein, healthy carbohydrates, and a variety of vegetables.

Lean beef: Choosing lean cuts of beef, such as sirloin or tenderloin, provides high-quality protein, iron, and other essential nutrients. Trim off any visible fat to reduce saturated fat content.

Stir-fry vegetables: Including a colorful assortment of vegetables in your stir-fry provides a wide range of antioxidants, vitamins, and minerals. Some great options are broccoli, carrots, bell peppers, snap peas, and mushrooms.

Brown rice: Opting for whole grains like brown rice instead of white rice provides more fiber, vitamins, and minerals. Brown rice retains its bran and germ layers, which are removed during the processing of white rice.

Example: A balanced lean beef stir-fry could include thinly-sliced lean beef cooked with a variety of colorful vegetables in a sauce made from low-sodium soy sauce, garlic, ginger, and a touch of honey. Serve over a portion of cooked brown rice.

Dessert: Frozen Yogurt

Enjoying a balanced dessert can be a guilt-free way to satisfy your sweet tooth while still providing some nutritional value. Frozen yogurt is a healthier alternative to traditional ice cream and can be enjoyed in moderation.

Frozen yogurt: Compared to ice cream, frozen yogurt typically has less fat and fewer calories. Look for options with live active cultures, which provide gut-friendly probiotics.

Toppings: When it comes to toppings, choose a variety of fresh fruits or a sprinkle of nuts for added nutrients and crunch. Avoid excessive amounts of high-sugar syrups or toppings.

Example: A balanced dessert could consist of a small serving of frozen yogurt, topped with a mix of fresh berries (such as strawberries, blueberries, or raspberries) and a sprinkle of crushed almonds.

Creating a Balanced Day

By focusing on the example meals and snacks provided, you can create your own balanced day of eating. Remember to incorporate a variety of food groups, choose whole, minimally processed foods, and pay attention to portion sizes. It's also essential to listen to your body's cues of hunger and fullness.

This guide has emphasized the importance of having a balanced day, starting with a wholesome breakfast, incorporating well-rounded snacks, and finishing with a satisfying dinner and dessert. Following these principles and making conscious choices can help you nourish your body while enjoying a wide variety of flavors and ingredients.

Tips for Long-Term Success

Long-term success in health and lifestyle changes necessitates a comprehensive approach encompassing diet, exercise, self-care, and behavior modification. By focusing on portion control and mindful eating, regular exercise and physical activity, staying hydrated, and managing stress and sleep, individuals can cultivate habits conducive to sustainability. This deep exploration elaborates on each aspect with examples, outlining their role in achieving enduring success.

Portion Control and Mindful Eating

The concept of portion control is pivotal for maintaining a healthy weight and nutrition. Portion control doesn't merely reduce calorie intake; it's a form of self-discipline that helps individuals avoid overindulgence, teaching the body to feel satisfied with enough food rather than an excess.

Example: Consider the Dietary Guidelines for Americans, which suggest filling half your plate with fruits and vegetables, a quarter with lean protein, and a quarter with whole grains. If someone typically eats a large plate full of pasta for dinner, they could adjust by serving themselves a smaller portion of pasta, adding a side salad, and some grilled chicken. This balanced approach can lead individuals to consume fewer calories while increasing nutrient intake.

Mindful eating goes hand-in-hand with portion control. It involves paying close attention to the experience of eating, the tastes, textures, and sensations, as well as recognizing hunger and fullness cues.

Example: When Lisa switched from eating lunch at her desk while working to sitting in the break room and focusing on her meal, she started to notice her hunger cues better. She began to eat slowly, savor the flavors, and found that she ate less and felt more satisfied because she was paying attention to her food rather than her work.

Regular Exercise and Physical Activity

Physical activity is a cornerstone of a healthy lifestyle. It doesn't need to be overly strenuous to be effective; consistently incorporating movement into one's daily routine can lead to major benefits over time.

Example: John started by walking 10 minutes each day. Eventually, as his fitness improved, he increased his walking time. Later, he began to include short jogging intervals. Over months, not only did his endurance improve, but his habit was firmly established.

In the case of people with busy schedules, finding innovative ways to incorporate exercise into daily activities can make a huge difference.

Example: Marie, an office worker, made it a point to use the stairs instead of the elevator and stood up every hour to stretch or walk around. These small alterations added up and improved her well-being without needing to find extra time in her day.

Staying Hydrated

Hydration is not merely about quenching thirst; it's essential for maintaining bodily functions, including metabolism and temperature regulation. The amount of fluid needed can vary widely based on individual factors like activity level, climate, and overall health.

Example: Sarah noticed that by increasing her water intake, her afternoon fatigue decreased significantly. She also experienced fewer headaches, which she hadn't realized were related to her habit of drinking very little water throughout the day.

Moreover, thirst can often be mistaken for hunger, leading to overeating when the body actually needs fluids.

Example: Tom realized he would often reach for snacks when in actuality, he was dehydrated. By drinking a glass of water before reaching for food, he could better assess if he was truly hungry.

Managing Stress and Sleep

Stress management and quality sleep are often overlooked but are vital for long-term success in maintaining healthy habits.

Chronic stress can lead to emotional eating, increased fat storage, and a reduction in the ability to make healthy choices. Techniques such as deep breathing, meditation, and yoga have been shown to be effective ways to manage stress.

Example: When Emily felt overwhelmed at work, she took five minutes to practice deep breathing exercises, which helped her manage her response to stress, reducing her inclination to grab comfort food.

Similarly, sleep is crucial as it affects hormones related to hunger and satiety. Lack of sleep can increase cravings for high-calorie foods.

Example: When Mark made an effort to get an extra hour of sleep each night, he not only saw improvements in his mood and cognitive function but he also experienced fewer cravings for unhealthy snacks throughout his day.

Practical Example: A comprehensive example of how these principles can combine to yield long-term success is the story of Alex. Alex wanted to improve his overall health and decided to tackle his goal from all four angles.

For portion control and mindful eating, Alex began using smaller plates to naturally reduce his portion sizes and made a rule to eat only at the dining table, free from distractions like TV or smartphones. He started listening to his body's cues for hunger and fullness and realized that he often ate out of boredom rather than true hunger, which led to unnecessary snacking.

To incorporate regular exercise, Alex initially started with a short walk during his lunch break and gradually added a morning routine of bodyweight exercises. This not only improved his physical strength and cardiovascular health but also enhanced his energy levels throughout the day.

For hydration, Alex kept a water bottle at his desk and set reminders to take sips regularly. He noticed a marked improvement in his concentration and a decrease in the mid-afternoon slump. He also began drinking a glass of water before meals, which helped with portion control.

In managing stress and sleep, Alex was proactive. He established a bedtime routine that included reading and light stretching, which helped him wind down from his day and prepare for a restful night's sleep. He also allocated time on weekends for hobbies that helped manage his stress levels, such as painting and hiking.

Six months into these lifestyle changes, Alex found that his efforts paid off. Not only had he lost weight, but he also felt more energized, focused, and in control of his health. His habits had changed in a way that felt natural and sustainable, providing a strong foundation for long-term success.

In conclusion, long-term success doesn't hinge on drastic measures or quick fixes. It's the small, consistent changes made day after day that become powerful over time. Portion control and mindful eating encourage a balanced approach to food intake. Regular exercise, even in small increments, can build fitness and improve health cumulatively. Adequate hydration supports overall well-being and aids in weight management. Finally, stress management and quality sleep are essential for allowing the body to recover and for maintaining the mental fortitude needed for these lifestyle changes. By weaving these strands together, individuals craft a resilient tapestry of habits that can support personal growth and health longevity.

Breakfast diet food Recipes

Starting your day with a healthy breakfast can give you the energy to keep going throughout the morning and help with better eating habits. Here's a list of 10 morning diet foods along with simple recipes you can incorporate into your morning routine.

1. Greek Yogurt Parfait
   Ingredients:
   - 1 cup Greek yogurt
   - 1/2 cup mixed berries (strawberries, blueberries, raspberries)
   - 2 tablespoons granola
   - 1 tablespoon honey (optional)

Preparation:
   Layer the Greek yogurt with berries and granola in a glass. Drizzle with honey if desired.

2. Oatmeal With Fruit and Nuts
   Ingredients:
   - 1/2 cup rolled oats
   - 1 cup water or milk
   - 1/2 banana, sliced
   - 1 tablespoon chopped almonds

- Cinnamon to taste
- Honey (optional)

Preparation:

Cook oatmeal as per the package directions using water or milk. Top with banana slices, almonds, cinnamon, and a drizzle of honey.

3. Avocado Toast
   Ingredients:
   - 1 slice whole grain bread
   - 1/2 ripe avocado
   - Salt and pepper to taste
   - Red pepper flakes (optional)
   - 1 poached or fried egg (optional)

Preparation:

Toast the bread and mash the avocado on top. Season with salt, pepper, and red pepper flakes. Add an egg on top for extra protein if desired.

4. Spinach and Feta Omelet
   Ingredients:
   - 2 eggs
   - Handful of fresh spinach leaves
   - 1/4 cup feta cheese, crumbled
   - 1/2 tablespoon olive oil

Preparation:

Heat olive oil in a pan, sauté spinach until wilted, beat the eggs and pour over the spinach, sprinkle feta cheese on top, and cook the omelet until the eggs are set.

5. Peanut Butter Banana Smoothie
   Ingredients:
   - 1 banana
   - 2 tablespoons peanut butter
   - 1 cup almond milk
   - Ice cubes (optional)

Preparation:
   Blend all ingredients until smooth.

6. Apple Cinnamon Quinoa Bowl
   Ingredients:
   - 1/2 cup cooked quinoa
   - 1 apple, diced
   - 1/2 teaspoon cinnamon
   - 1 tablespoon walnuts, chopped
   - Honey or maple syrup (optional)

Preparation:
   Mix warm quinoa with diced apple, cinnamon, and walnuts.
Sweeten with honey or maple syrup if desired.

7. Chia Seed Pudding
   Ingredients:
   - 1/4 cup chia seeds
   - 1 cup almond milk
   - 1 tablespoon honey or maple syrup
   - 1/2 teaspoon vanilla extract (optional)
   - Fresh berries for topping

Preparation:

Mix chia seeds, almond milk, sweetener, and vanilla in a bowl. Refrigerate for at least 2 hours or overnight, until it forms a pudding-like consistency. Top with fresh berries.

8. Turkey and Cheese Roll-ups
   Ingredients:
   - Sliced turkey breast
   - Sliced cheese of your choice
   - Whole grain tortilla or lettuce leaves

Preparation:

Place turkey and cheese on a tortilla or a lettuce leaf and roll it up. You can add mustard or hummus for extra flavor.

9. Multigrain Pancakes
   Ingredients:
   - 1 cup multigrain pancake mix
   - 1 cup water or milk
   - Fresh fruit or berries (optional)

Preparation:

Prepare the pancake batter according to package instructions and cook pancakes on a hot griddle. Serve with fresh fruit or berries on top.

10. Cottage Cheese With Pineapple
    Ingredients:
    - 1/2 cup cottage cheese
    - 1/2 cup pineapple chunks (fresh or canned in juice)

Preparation:

Mix cottage cheese with pineapple chunks for a sweet and savory breakfast.

40

These are just a few ideas for nutritious breakfasts that can help set a healthy tone for your day. Adjust portion sizes and ingredients according to your dietary needs and preferences. Remember, drinking water in the morning is also important for rehydration and kickstarting your metabolism.

Lunch diet food Recipes

Certainly! Below are ten lunch diet food recipes, each with a list of ingredients. Keep in mind that "diet food" can mean different things to different people, so I've included a variety of healthy, nutrient-rich options. Always adjust portions and ingredients to suit your specific dietary needs and preferences.

1. Chicken Salad with Mixed Greens
   - Cooked chicken breast (chopped or shredded)
   - Mixed salad greens (spinach, arugula, lettuce)
   - Cherry tomatoes, halved
   - Cucumber, sliced
   - Red onion, thinly sliced
   - Avocado, cubed
   - Olive oil
   - Lemon juice or balsamic vinegar
   - Salt and pepper to taste

2. Quinoa and Black Bean Bowl
   - Cooked quinoa
   - Black beans (rinsed and drained if from a can)
   - Corn kernels
   - Red bell pepper, diced
   - Cilantro, chopped
   - Lime juice

- Chili powder
- Cumin
- Salt and pepper to taste

3. Greek Yogurt and Berry Parfait
    - Greek yogurt (unsweetened)
    - Mixed berries (strawberries, blueberries, raspberries)
    - A drizzle of honey (optional)
    - Chopped nuts (almonds, walnuts, or pistachios)
    - Ground flaxseed or chia seeds

4. Turkey and Hummus Wrap
    - Whole grain or low-carb wrap
    - Sliced turkey breast (low sodium)
    - Hummus
    - Spinach or lettuce leaves
    - Sliced cucumber
    - Sliced tomato
    - Sliced red onion
    - Salt and pepper to taste

5. Zucchini Noodle Salad
    - Zucchini, spiralized into noodles
    - Cherry tomatoes, halved
    - Olives, sliced
    - Feta cheese, crumbled
    - Olive oil
    - Lemon juice
    - Garlic, minced
    - Fresh basil, chopped
    - Salt and pepper to taste

6. Tuna and White Bean Salad
   - Canned tuna in water, drained
   - White beans (cannellini or Great Northern), rinsed and drained
   - Red onion, finely chopped
   - Parsley, chopped
   - Olive oil
   - Lemon juice
   - Salt and cracked black pepper to taste

7. Grilled Vegetable and Feta Salad
   - Zucchini, sliced lengthwise
   - Bell peppers, sliced
   - Eggplant, sliced
   - Red onion, wedges
   - Olive oil
   - Balsamic vinegar
   - Fresh basil or thyme
   - Feta cheese, crumbled
   - Salt and pepper to taste

8. Asian Chicken Lettuce Wraps
   - Ground chicken breast
   - Garlic, minced
   - Fresh ginger, grated
   - Low-sodium soy sauce or tamari
   - Sesame oil
   - Sriracha or chili flakes (optional for spice)
   - Carrot, grated
   - Water chestnuts, chopped
   - Green onions, sliced

- Lettuce leaves (such as Bibb or iceberg)

9. Lentil Soup
    - Green or brown lentils, rinsed
    - Carrot, diced
    - Celery, diced
    - Onion, diced
    - Garlic, minced
    - Low-sodium vegetable or chicken broth
    - Diced tomatoes (canned)
    - Bay leaves
    - Olive oil
    - Cumin
    - Thyme
    - Salt and pepper to taste

10. Spinach and Egg White Omelette
    - Egg whites
    - Fresh spinach leaves
    - Mushrooms, sliced
    - Red bell pepper, diced
    - Onion, diced
    - Low-fat cheese (optional)
    - Salt and pepper to taste
    - Cooking spray or a small amount of oil for the pan

These recipes are focused on using whole foods and aiming for balanced nutrition to support a healthy diet. You can adjust the ingredients and their quantities to match your dietary goals, such as low-carb, high-protein, Mediterranean-style, or vegetarian diets. Enjoy your healthy lunches!

Dinner diet food Recipes

Certainly! When it comes to dinner recipes that are diet-friendly, the goal is usually to find meals that are nutritious, satisfying, and low in calories. Here are 10 recipes that fit those criteria:

1. Grilled Chicken Salad
   Ingredients:
   - 2 grilled chicken breasts (skinless)
   - Mixed salad greens
   - Cherry tomatoes
   - Cucumber, sliced
   - Red onion, thinly sliced
   - Balsamic vinaigrette

Instructions:

1. Grill the chicken breasts until fully cooked and slice them.
2. Combine the salad greens, cherry tomatoes, cucumber, and red onion in a large bowl.
3. Top with the sliced chicken and drizzle with balsamic vinaigrette before serving.

2. Steamed Fish with Vegetables
   Ingredients:

- 2 white fish fillets (like tilapia or cod)
- Mixed vegetables (e.g., broccoli, carrots, bell peppers)
- Lemon juice
- Fresh herbs (like dill or parsley)
- Salt and pepper to taste

Instructions:

1. Season the fish with lemon juice, salt, and pepper.
2. Steam the fish and vegetables until the fish is flaky and vegetables are tender, about 5-7 minutes.
3. Garnish with fresh herbs and serve immediately.

3. Quinoa and Black Bean Bowl
   Ingredients:
   - 1 cup cooked quinoa
   - 1 cup black beans, cooked and drained
   - Cherry tomatoes, halved
   - Avocado, sliced
   - Fresh cilantro, chopped
   - Lime wedges

Instructions:

1. In a bowl, layer cooked quinoa with black beans and cherry tomatoes.
2. Top with sliced avocado and chopped cilantro.
3. Squeeze lime over the bowl before serving.

4. Sautéed Shrimp with Zucchini Noodles
   Ingredients:
   - Shrimp, peeled and deveined
   - Zucchini, spiralized into noodles
   - Garlic, minced
   - Olive oil
   - Chili flakes (optional)
   - Salt and pepper to taste

Instructions:

   1. Heat olive oil in a pan and sauté garlic until fragrant.
   2. Add the shrimp and cook until pink and opaque.
   3. Toss in zucchini noodles and cook until just tender.
   4. Season with chili flakes, salt, and pepper, then serve.

5. Turkey and Vegetable Stir-Fry
   Ingredients:
   - Ground turkey
   - Mixed vegetables (e.g., broccoli, bell peppers, and mushrooms)
   - Soy sauce (or tamari for gluten-free)
   - Garlic, minced
   - Ginger, minced
   - Olive oil

Instructions:

   1. Heat olive oil in a pan and brown the ground turkey.
   2. Add garlic, ginger, and vegetables and stir-fry until veg-

etables are cooked yet crisp.

3. Toss with soy sauce and serve over brown rice if desired.

6. Lentil Soup

Ingredients:
- Lentils, rinsed and drained
- Carrots, diced
- Celery, diced
- Onion, diced
- Vegetable broth
- Diced tomatoes
- Garlic, minced
- Seasonings: bay leaf, thyme, salt, and pepper

Instructions:

1. In a pot, sauté onions, garlic, carrots, and celery.
2. Add the lentils, broth, tomatoes, and seasonings.
3. Bring to a boil, then simmer until lentils are soft.
4. Serve hot, garnished with fresh herbs if available.

7. Roasted Cauliflower Steaks

Ingredients:
- Cauliflower, sliced into thick steaks
- Olive oil
- Garlic powder
- Paprika
- Salt and pepper to taste

Instructions:

1. Preheat the oven to 425°F (220°C).
2. Brush cauliflower steaks with olive oil and season with garlic powder, paprika, salt, and pepper.
3. Roast until tender and golden, about 20-25 minutes.

8. Greek Salad with Tofu Feta
   Ingredients:
   - Mixed greens
   - Cherry tomatoes, halved
   - Cucumber, sliced
   - Red onion, thinly sliced
   - Kalamata olives
   - Tofu, pressed and crumbled
   - Lemon juice
   - Olive oil
   - Oregano

Instructions:

1. For tofu feta, marinate crumbled tofu in lemon juice, olive oil, and oregano for at least 30 minutes.
2. Combine salad ingredients in a bowl.
3. Top with tofu feta and serve with a drizzle of olive oil and vinegar if desired.

9. Baked Salmon with Asparagus
   Ingredients:

- Salmon fillets
- Asparagus, trimmed
- Lemon slices
- Olive oil
- Salt and pepper to taste

Instructions:

1. Preheat the oven to 400°F (200°C).
2. Place salmon and asparagus on a baking sheet.
3. Drizzle with olive oil and season with salt and pepper.
4. Top with lemon slices and bake for around 12–15 minutes.

10. Spaghetti Squash Primavera
Ingredients:
- Spaghetti squash, halved and seeds removed
- Assorted vegetables (e.g., bell peppers, onions, zucchini)
- Marinara sauce
- Garlic, minced
- Olive oil
- Basil, chopped
- Grated Parmesan cheese (optional)

Instructions:

1. Roast spaghetti squash in the oven at 400°F (200°C) until tender, about 45 minutes.
2. Sauté garlic and vegetables in olive oil until just tender.
3. Scrape out the spaghetti squash strands and toss with vegetables and marinara sauce.

4. Garnish with fresh basil and Parmesan before serving.

Remember that portion control is key for a diet-friendly meal, so adjust the serving sizes to your dietary needs. Additionally, consider the nutritional goals of your specific diet when selecting recipes, as some may focus on low-carb, low-fat, high-protein, or other specific requirements.

www.ingramcontent.com/pod-product-compliance
Lightning Source LLC
Chambersburg PA
CBHW071110260726

48661CB00006B/2566